WALL PILATES FOR MEN

Low-Impact And Gentle Exercises For Beginners And Seniors To Build Strength, Flexibility And Core Stability

Randy T. Lucas

Copyright 2023, Randy T. Lucas

Table of Contents

INTRODUCTION

In the hustle and bustle of modern life, finding a workout routine that harmonizes strength, flexibility, and mindfulness can feel like discovering a hidden oasis. Meet John – a dedicated professional juggling the demands of work and family life. For years, he struggled to find a fitness regimen that complemented his hectic schedule and provided holistic well-being. Then, he stumbled upon Wall Pilates.

With skepticism initially clouding his thoughts about this seemingly unconventional approach, John decided to explore. Little did he know that embracing Wall Pilates would transform his fitness journey. Within weeks of integrating this innovative method into his routine, he felt a surge of strength ripple through his muscles, noticed increased flexibility, and experienced a newfound sense of balance.

Driven by the desire to share this transformative experience, John embarked on a quest to delve deeper into the world of Wall Pilates, understanding its core principles, and crafting a tailored guide specifically for men.

Introduction: Embracing Wall Pilates for Men

Welcome to the world of Wall Pilates, a unique fusion of strength, flexibility, and mindfulness exercises tailored to meet the distinct needs of men. In a fitness landscape often dominated by high-impact workouts and muscle-pumping routines, Wall Pilates offers a refreshing alternative – a holistic approach that doesn't just sculpt the body but nurtures it from within.

This guide aims to introduce men to the incredible benefits of Wall Pilates, a versatile and effective workout method that utilizes the support of a wall to enhance movements, deepen stretches, and refine postures. Whether you're a beginner seeking an entry point into mindful fitness or a seasoned athlete aiming to diversify your routine, Wall Pilates for Men is designed to cater to your individual needs.

Discover the Essence of Wall Pilates

At its core, Wall Pilates combines elements of Pilates, yoga, and functional training, emphasizing controlled movements, proper alignment, and breath awareness. By leveraging the stability of a wall, individuals engage muscles more efficiently, allowing for a deeper connection and activation of the body's powerhouse – the core muscles.

The journey through this guide will unravel a series of exercises meticulously crafted to target specific areas of the body from enhancing upper body strength to fortifying the core and improving lower body flexibility and stability.

What to Expect

Each section of this guide is intricately curated to offer step-by-step instructions, accompanied by illustrative visuals, ensuring a clear understanding of every exercise. Additionally, safety tips, progressions, and advanced techniques will be shared to assist in your evolution within the practice of Wall Pilates.

So, whether you're seeking to alleviate back pain, enhance posture, or simply amplify your overall fitness, allow this guide to be your gateway into the transformative world of Wall Pilates designed exclusively for men.

CHAPTER 1

Understanding Wall Pilates for Men

What is Wall Pilates?

Wall Pilates is a dynamic exercise methodology that integrates principles from Pilates, yoga, and functional training, utilizing a wall for support, stability, and enhanced movement precision. Tailored specifically for men, this practice emphasizes controlled movements, proper alignment, and breath awareness to strengthen muscles, improve flexibility, and promote overall well-being.

Key Elements of Wall Pilates for Men

1. Controlled Movements: Each exercise focuses on deliberate and controlled movements to engage specific muscle groups effectively.

2. Core Activation: Wall Pilates places a strong emphasis on engaging and strengthening the core muscles, which are essential for stability and overall strength.

3. Breath Awareness: Conscious breathing is an integral part of Wall Pilates, aiding in movement coordination and enhancing mind-body connection.

Benefits of Wall Pilates for Men

1. Enhanced Core Strength: Targeted exercises fortify abdominal muscles, promoting core stability and strength crucial for posture and overall functionality.

2. Improved Flexibility: Through stretching and controlled movements, Wall Pilates enhances flexibility, reducing the risk of injuries and increasing range of motion.

3. Muscle Tone and Definition: Consistent practice leads to well-defined and toned muscles, especially in the core, arms, legs, and back.

4. Better Posture: Strengthening core muscles aids in maintaining proper posture, alleviating back pain and improving overall spinal alignment.

5. Increased Body Awareness: Wall Pilates emphasizes mind-body connection, promoting greater awareness of body alignment and movement patterns.

6. Enhanced Balance and Stability: Exercises targeting balance and stability improve coordination and functional movement.

7. Injury Prevention: Strengthening muscles and enhancing flexibility can reduce the risk of injury during physical activities or daily movements.

8. Stress Reduction: Mindful breathing techniques incorporated in Wall Pilates help reduce stress and promote relaxation.

9. Better Athletic Performance: Improved core strength, flexibility, and body control translate into enhanced athletic performance in various sports and activities.

10. Adaptability and Accessibility: Wall Pilates routines can be adapted to varying fitness levels and are accessible for individuals of different ages and abilities.

10 Safety Tips and Precautions for Wall Pilates

1. Consult a Professional: Before starting any exercise program, consult a healthcare provider or fitness professional, especially if you have pre-existing medical conditions.

2. Warm-up: Always warm up before starting Wall Pilates to prepare your body for exercise.

3. Proper Form: Focus on maintaining proper form and alignment during each exercise to prevent injury.

4. Start Slowly: Begin with easier exercises and slowly progress to more advanced movements as your strength and flexibility improve.

5. Listen to Your Body: Pay attention to your body's signals and avoid pushing beyond your limits.

6. Use Props Carefully: If incorporating props or equipment, ensure they are used correctly and safely.

7. Breath Control: Coordinate your breath with movements to optimize effectiveness and prevent breath-holding.

8. Hydration: Stay hydrated throughout your workout session.

9. Rest and Recovery: Allow adequate time for rest and recovery between workout sessions to prevent overexertion.

10. Modify as Needed: If an exercise causes discomfort or pain, modify or skip it and seek guidance from a fitness professional.

CHAPTER 2

Upper Body Workouts

Shoulder Stretches and Exercises

1. Wall Angels:

- Place your feet hip-width apart and lean your back against the wall.

- Lift your arms to shoulder height, bending them at the elbows so that they are in a goal-post position, palms facing forward.

- Slowly slide your arms up the wall as high as comfortable, maintaining contact with the wall.

- Hold for a moment, then slowly lower your arms back to the starting position. Repeat for 10-12 reps.

2. Shoulder Blade Squeeze:

- Stand or sit tall with your back against the wall and your arms by your sides.

- Engage your core and gently squeeze your shoulder blades together, imagining you're trying to hold a pencil between them.

- Hold it for 5-10 seconds, then release. Repeat for 12-15 repetitions.

3. Shoulder Circles:

- Stand tall, feet shoulder-width apart, and extend your arms out to the sides at shoulder height.

- Start making small circular motions with your arms, rotating your shoulders backward.

- Gradually increase the size of the circles, aiming for a full range of motion. After 10 circles backward, switch to 10 circles forward.

Arm Strengthening with Wall Resistance

1. Wall Push-Ups:

- Stand facing the wall, arms extended at shoulder height and hands flat against the wall, slightly wider than shoulder-width apart.

- Bend your elbows to bring your chest closer to the wall while maintaining a straight body from head to heels.

- Push back to the starting position by straightening your arms. Aim for 10-15 repetitions.

2. Wall Tricep Dips:

- Sit on the floor with your back against the wall and your hands placed behind you, shoulder-width apart on the floor, fingers pointing towards your body.

- Lift your hips off the ground and walk your feet forward, supporting your weight on your hands and heels.

- Bend your elbows to lower your body toward the floor, then straighten your arms to return to the starting position. Repeat for 12-15 reps.

3. Wall Bicep Curls:

- Stand facing the wall, with your feet about a foot away from it.

- Place your hands against the wall at shoulder height, palms flat.

- Slowly bend your elbows, bringing your chest closer to the wall, then push back to the starting position. Perform 12-15 repetitions.

Chest and Upper Back Engagements

1. Wall Chest Press:

- Stand facing away from the wall and extend your arms backward to shoulder height, palms flat against the wall.
- Bend your elbows to bring your chest closer to the wall, then push back to the starting position. Aim for 10-12 reps.

2. Wall Rows:

- Stand facing the wall, arms extended at chest height, palms against the wall.
- Pull your body towards the wall by bending your elbows, keeping them close to your sides, then return to the starting position. Repeat for 10-12 repetitions.

3. Wall Shoulder Blade Squeeze and Hold:

- Stand with your back against the wall and your arms extended out to the sides at shoulder height, palms facing forward.

- Squeeze your shoulder blades together while maintaining contact with the wall.

- Hold the squeeze for 10-15 seconds, then relax. Repeat for 3-4 sets.

These exercises can be incorporated into a comprehensive Upper Body workout routine focusing on shoulder stretches, arm strengthening with wall resistance, and engagements targeting the chest and upper back muscles in your 'Wall Pilates for Men' guide.

CHAPTER 3

Core Strengthening

Abdominal Exercises using the Wall

1. Wall Plank:

- With your feet against the wall and your hands shoulder-width apart on the floor, begin in the plank position with your back to the wall.

- Maintain a straight line from head to heels, engaging your core muscles.

- Hold the position for 30 seconds to 1 minute, gradually increasing duration with practice.

2. Wall Knee Tucks:

- Starting with your feet on the wall and your hands on the floor, assume a plank position facing the wall.

- Bring your knees to your chest by using your core, then extend them back to their initial position. Aim for twelve to fifteen reps.

3. Wall Sit-Ups:

- Lie on your back with your legs extended vertically against the wall, forming a 90-degree angle with your body.

- Perform sit-ups by lifting your upper body towards your knees, engaging your abdominal muscles. Aim for 10-12 reps.

Oblique Workouts and Rotational Movements

1. Side Plank with Leg Lift:

- Start in a side plank position, placing your feet on the wall or stacking them one in front of the other, with your forearm on the floor.

- Lift your top leg towards the ceiling, engaging your obliques.

- Hold for 15-30 seconds, then switch sides. Aim for 3 sets on each side.

2. Russian Twists with Wall Support:

- Sit on the floor with your knees bent, feet against the wall, and lean back slightly, keeping your back straight.

- Hold a weighted object (e.g., a medicine ball or dumbbell) and rotate your torso from side to side, touching the object to the ground near your hip. Aim for 12-15 twists on each side.

3. Wall Knee-to-Elbow Twists:

- Begin with your feet up against the wall and your hands on the floor, facing away from the wall in a plank posture.

- Alternately bring each knee towards the opposite elbow in a twisting motion, engaging your obliques. Aim for 10-12 repetitions on each side.

Lower Back Support and Strengthening

1. Wall Superman:

- Lie face down on the floor with your feet against the wall and arms extended overhead.

- Lift your chest, arms, and legs off the ground, engaging your lower back muscles, and hold the position for 15-30 seconds. Repeat for 3 sets.

2. Wall Bridge:

- Lay flat on your back with your knees bent 90 degrees and your feet resting against the wall.

- Lift your hips off the ground, creating a straight line from shoulders to knees. Hold for 15-30 seconds and release. Aim for 3 sets.

3. Wall Cat-Cow Stretch:

- Kneel facing the wall and place your hands on the wall at shoulder height.

- Arch your back, pushing away from the wall (cow position), then round your spine towards the wall (cat position). Repeat this fluid movement for 10-12 repetitions.

Incorporate these exercises into your 'Wall Pilates for Men' guide to create a well-rounded core-strengthening routine focusing on abdominal exercises, oblique workouts, rotational movements, and lower back support and strengthening.

CHAPTER 4

Lower Body Engagements

Wall Squats and Leg Strengthening

1. Wall Squats:

- Place your feet hip-width apart and lean back against the wall.

- Slide down the wall, bending your knees until they form a 90-degree angle. Keep your back against the wall and thighs parallel to the floor.

- Hold this position for 30 seconds to 1 minute, gradually increasing the duration as you build strength.

2. Wall Sit Leg Raises:

- Begin in a wall squat position with your thighs parallel to the floor.

- While maintaining the squat, lift one leg straight out in front of you, hold for a few seconds, then lower it back down. Alternate legs and aim for 10-12 raises on each leg.

3. Wall Lunges:

- Stand about 2 feet away from the wall, facing away from it.

- Step back with one leg and place your foot against the wall, lowering your body into a lunge position. Push back to the starting position. Alternate legs and perform 10-12 lunges on each side.

Hamstring Stretches and Flexibility

1. Wall Hamstring Stretch:

- Lie on your back with your hips close to the wall and legs extended upward, resting against the wall.

- Slowly walk your hands down your legs towards your feet, gently pulling your legs closer to your body until you feel a stretch in your hamstrings. Hold for 30 seconds to 1 minute.

2. Wall Supported Forward Fold:

- Stand facing the wall, a few feet away from it.

- Lean forward and place your hands against the wall at shoulder height. Walk your hands down the wall as you hinge at your hips, keeping your back straight, until you feel a stretch in your hamstrings. Hold for 30 seconds.

3. Wall Runner's Stretch:

- Face the wall and extend one leg straight behind you, placing the heel on the ground.

- Lean forward, keeping your hands on the wall for support, until you feel a stretch in your rear leg's hamstring. Hold for 30 seconds and switch legs.

Calf Muscles Exercises against the Wall

1. Wall Calf Raises:

- Stand facing the wall with your hands resting against it at shoulder height.

- Rise onto the balls of your feet, lifting your heels very high, then lower them back down. Aim for 15-20 repetitions.

2. Wall Calf Stretch:

- Stand arm's length away from the wall and place your hands against it at shoulder height.

- Step one foot back and press the heel into the ground, keeping the back leg straight and feeling the stretch in your calf. Hold for 30 seconds and switch legs.

3. Wall Calf Raises with Eccentric Lowering:

- Stand facing the wall with your hands resting against it for support.

- Rise onto the balls of your feet, lift your heels, and then slowly lower them back down, taking at least 3-4 seconds to complete the lowering phase. Repeat for 12-15 repetitions.

Integrate these exercises into your 'Wall Pilates for Men' guide to create a comprehensive lower body engagement routine focusing on wall squats, hamstring stretches, flexibility, and calf muscle exercises against the wall.

CHAPTER 5

Whole Body Integration

Full Body Wall Pilates Flow

1. Wall Roll-Down to Roll-Up:

- Stand with your back against the wall, feet hip-width apart.

- Slowly roll your spine down, articulating each vertebra, until your hands touch the floor. Hold for a moment.

- Roll back up to standing, sequentially stacking each vertebra. Repeat for 8-10 reps.

2. Wall Squat with Arm Reaches:

- Perform a wall squat with your back against the wall and thighs parallel to the floor.

- As you hold the squat, lift your arms overhead, then lower them back down to shoulder height. Alternate reaching arms while maintaining the squat position. Aim for 10-12 reaches on each side.

3. Wall Plank with Alternating Leg Lifts:

- Assume a plank position facing the wall, hands on the floor, and feet against the wall.

- Lift one leg off the wall, extending it straight back, then return to the starting position. Alternate legs and perform 10-12 lifts on each side.

Integrating Upper, Core, and Lower Body Movements

1. Wall Mountain Climbers:

- Begin in a plank position facing the wall, hands on the floor and feet against the wall.

- Alternately drive your knees towards your chest in a running motion, engaging your core. Aim for 20-30 mountain climbers (10-15 per leg).

2. Wall Push-Up to Knee Tuck:

- Start in a push-up position facing the wall, hands on the floor and feet against the wall.

- Perform a push-up, then bring one knee towards your chest in a tucking motion. Alternate legs and aim for 10-12 repetitions (5-6 per leg).

3. Wall Side Plank with Arm Reach:

- Assume a side plank position with your forearm on the floor and feet against the wall, stacking your feet or one in front of the other.

- Lift your top arm towards the ceiling, then reach under your body, threading it between your torso and the wall. Return to the starting position. Aim for 8-10 reaches on each side.

Balance and Stability Exercises using the Wall

1. Wall Single-Leg Balance:

- Stand near the wall and lift one leg off the ground, balancing on the other.

- Hold the position for 20-30 seconds, then switch legs. Repeat for 3 sets on each leg.

2. Wall Knee Lifts with Rotation:

- Stand sideways to the wall, using one hand for support.

- Lift the outside knee towards your chest, then rotate your torso, bringing the knee towards the opposite elbow. Repeat for 10-12 lifts on each side.

3. Wall Supported Warrior III:

- Face the wall and place your hands against it at shoulder height.

- Lift one leg straight behind you while leaning forward, creating a T-shape with your body. Hold for 15-20 seconds and switch legs.

Incorporate these exercises into your 'Wall Pilates for Men' guide to create a well-balanced whole-body integration routine focusing on full-body flows, integration of upper, core, and lower body movements, as well as balance and stability exercises using the wall.

CHAPTER 6

Advanced Techniques

Progressions and Advanced Wall Pilates Movements

1. Wall Pike Press:

- Begin in a plank position facing the wall, hands on the floor and feet against the wall.

- Walk your hands closer to the wall, lifting your hips and forming an inverted V shape. Perform push-ups in this position, aiming for 8-10 reps.

2. Wall Walks:

- Begin with your feet up against the wall and your hands on the floor, facing away from the wall in a plank posture.

- Walk your feet up the wall while walking your hands closer to the wall, eventually reaching a near-vertical position. Slowly walk back down. Repeat for 3-4 walks.

3. Wall Handstand Hold:

- Face the wall, kick up into a handstand with your feet resting against the wall for support.

- Aim to hold the handstand position against the wall for 20-30 seconds, gradually increasing the duration as your strength improves.

Incorporating Props for Added Challenge

1. Medicine Ball Wall Squat Throws:

- Perform wall squats with your back against the wall while holding a medicine ball at chest height.

- As you rise from the squat, explosively throw the ball against the wall, catching it upon return. Aim for 10-12 throws.

2. Resistance Band Wall Pull-Aparts:

- Stand facing the wall and hold a resistance band with both hands at shoulder height.

- Pull the band apart, stretching it against the wall, then slowly return to the starting position. Perform 12-15 repetitions.

3. Bosu Ball Wall Plank with Leg Lifts:

- Place a Bosu ball on the floor against the wall and assume a plank position with your feet on the Bosu and hands on the floor.

- Lift one leg off the Bosu, extending it straight back, then return to the starting position. Aim for 10-12 lifts on each leg.

Customizing Wall Pilates Routines for Men

1. Progressive Routine Customization:

- Encourage men to gradually increase the intensity, duration, or complexity of exercises as they gain strength and proficiency in Wall Pilates.

2. Targeted Muscle Group Focus:

- Provide guidance on customizing routines to focus on specific muscle groups based on individual goals, such as emphasizing core work or upper body strength.

3. Time-Based Customization:

- Suggest options for customizing workouts based on time constraints, allowing for shorter, more intense sessions or longer, more comprehensive routines to suit varying schedules.

Integrate these advanced techniques into your 'Wall Pilates for Men' guide to offer progressive and challenging exercises, incorporating props for added difficulty, and providing insights on customizing Wall Pilates routines tailored specifically for men's fitness goals and preferences.

CONCLUSION

As we wrap up this guide on Wall Pilates specifically designed for men, it's like closing a chapter on a remarkable journey toward better health and fitness. Throughout this guide, we've explored how Wall Pilates isn't just about exercises, it's about connecting with our bodies, improving strength, flexibility, and finding a sense of balance in our busy lives.

Understanding the core principles of Wall Pilates has been like discovering the secret behind its magic. It's all about controlled movements, paying attention to our breath, and activating those core muscles for a stronger and more tuned-in body.

What's been truly exciting is uncovering the array of benefits this practice brings. From getting a stronger core to feeling more flexible and even relieving stress, Wall Pilates offers so much more than just a workout routine. It's a gateway to a better, more harmonious lifestyle.

Safety has been a top priority throughout this journey. We've walked through exercises, ensuring everyone stays safe while progressing. The emphasis has always been on listening to our bodies and avoiding overdoing it.

For those seeking an extra challenge, we've unveiled advanced techniques and prop-based exercises to push the boundaries. And we've talked about how recovery after a session is just as important, it's about stretching, taking care of those muscles, and ensuring a lasting commitment to fitness.

This guide isn't just about exercising; it's about living better. It's an invitation for guys to embrace a journey that doesn't just end here. It's about making Wall Pilates a part of life, a lifestyle choice that brings strength, balance, and a positive mindset.

So, as we say goodbye to this guide, it's more of a 'see you later' to the beginning of a healthier, more energized, and resilient future. Here's to embracing the transformative power of Wall Pilates and to all the incredible benefits it brings to men's lives. Cheers to a future filled with strength, balance, and an enduring commitment to wellness!

FITNESS

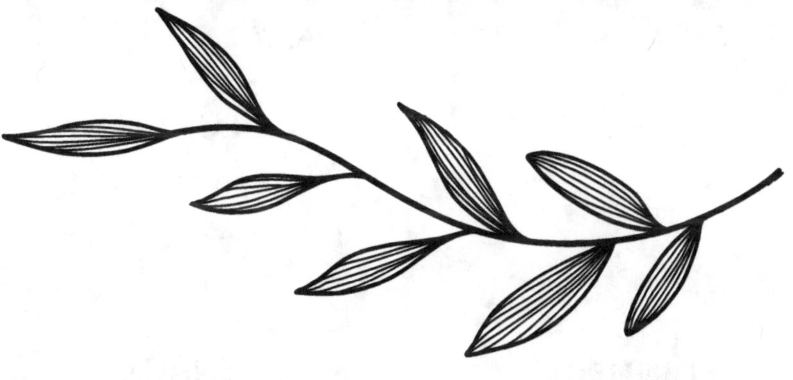

PLANNER

Fitness Planner

NAME: DATE:

BREAKFAST

LUNCH

DINNER

SNACK

EXERCISE	SET	REP	NOTES

Fitness Planner

NAME:

DATE:

BREAKFAST

LUNCH

DINNER

SNACK

EXERCISE

SET

REP

NOTES

Fitness Planner

NAME: DATE:

BREAKFAST

LUNCH

DINNER

SNACK

EXERCISE	SET	REP	NOTES

Fitness Planner

NAME:

DATE:

BREAKFAST

LUNCH

DINNER

SNACK

EXERCISE

SET

REP

NOTES

Fitness Planner

NAME: **DATE:**

BREAKFAST   ## LUNCH

DINNER   ## SNACK

EXERCISE   SET   REP   NOTES

Fitness Planner

NAME:

DATE:

BREAKFAST

LUNCH

DINNER

SNACK

EXERCISE

SET

REP

NOTES

Fitness Planner

NAME:

DATE:

BREAKFAST

LUNCH

DINNER

SNACK

EXERCISE	SET	REP	NOTES

Fitness Planner

NAME: DATE:

BREAKFAST   LUNCH

DINNER   SNACK

EXERCISE   SET   REP   NOTES

Fitness Planner

NAME: **DATE:**

BREAKFAST

LUNCH

DINNER

SNACK

EXERCISE	SET	REP	NOTES

Fitness Planner

NAME: DATE:

BREAKFAST   LUNCH

DINNER   SNACK

EXERCISE   SET   REP   NOTES

www.ingramcontent.com/pod-product-compliance
Lightning Source LLC
Chambersburg PA
CBHW071112260726
48661CB00006B/2582